THE OSTEOPOROSIS DIET COOKBOOK FOR WOMEN

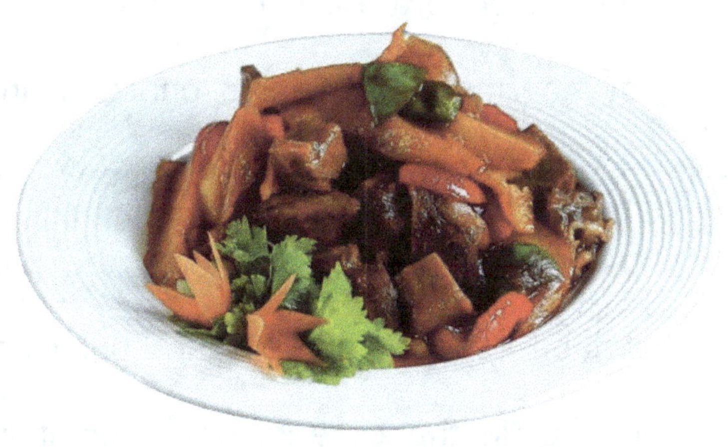

Flavorful Recipes for Stronger Bones and Healthier Lives

Dr. Samantha Hayes

TABLE OF CONTENTS

INTRODUCTION............................6

NOTE FROM THE AUTHOR.............6

CHAPTER 1...........................12

Understanding Osteoporosis...........12

What is Osteoporosis?.................12

Types of Osteoporosis.................15

Causes of Osteoporosis..............18

Symptoms of Osteoporosis.........23

Preventive Measures for Osteoporosis.................................26

Chapter 2.............................30

Importance of Nutrition in Managing Osteoporosis 30

Foods to Eat for Stronger Bones.....34

Foods to Avoid to Reduce Bone Loss 37

CHAPTER 3...........................42

Osteoporosis Diet Recipes.............42

Breakfast Recipes 42

1. Calcium-Rich Smoothie 42

2. Greek Yogurt Parfait with Berries and Almonds 44

3. Spinach and Mushroom Frittata 46

4. Avocado Toast with Poached Egg...48

5. Whole Grain Pancakes With Blueberries And Walnuts 50

6. Spinach and Feta Breakfast Wrap 52

7. Overnight Oats with Almond Butter and Banana 54

8. Veggie Breakfast Burrito 56

9. Cottage Cheese and Fruit Bowl 58

10. Quinoa Breakfast Bowl 59

Lunch Recipes...............................60

1. Grilled Salmon Salad 60

2. Quinoa Stuffed Bell peppers 62

3. Chicken and Vegetable Stir-Fry 64

4. Lentils and Vegetable Soup 66

5. Spinach and Mushroom Quesadilla 68

6. Turkey and Veggie Wrap 70

7. Chickpea Salad Sandwich 72

8. Spinach and Feta Turkey Burger 74

9. Veggie and Hummus Wrap......76

10. Mediterranean Chickpea Salad 78

Dinner Recipes 80

1. Baked Salmon with Roasted Vegetables 80

2. Quinoa and Black Bean Stuffed Peppers.......................................82

3. Chicken and Vegetable Skewers with Quinoa 84

4. Spinach and Feta Stuffed Chicken Breast............................86

5. Lentil and Vegetable Curry 88

6. Turkey and Vegetable Stir-Fry .90

7.   Spinach   and   Ricotta   Stuffed shells...92

8. Vegetable and Tofu Stir-Fry.....94

9. Baked Chicken Parmesan 96

10. Vegetable and Lentil Soup.....98

CONCLUSION…………………100

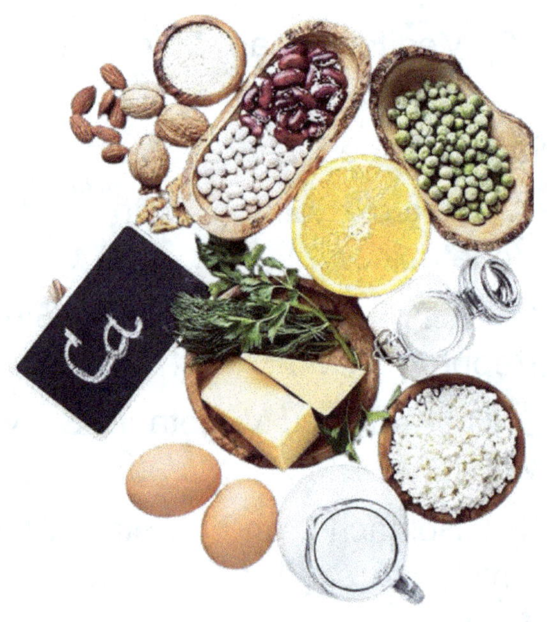

INTRODUCTION
NOTE FROM THE AUTHOR

Dear Reader,

As you delve into the chapters of this cookbook, I extend to you my heartfelt gratitude and warmest wishes on your journey towards better health and well-being. Within these pages, you will find not only a collection of delicious recipes but also a wealth of knowledge aimed at supporting your bone health and overall vitality.

My journey with osteoporosis began as a professional pursuit, woven intricately into the fabric of my medical career. As a dedicated physician, I have witnessed firsthand the profound impact that this condition can have on individuals and their loved ones. It is a silent adversary, often lurking in the shadows, yet its effects can be far-reaching and life-altering.

In my clinical practice, I have encountered countless patients grappling with the challenges posed by osteoporosis—individuals whose lives have been touched by fractures, pain, and the fear of what the future may hold. It is their stories, their resilience, and their unwavering determination that have inspired me to embark on this journey—to create a resource that empowers and educates, offering a beacon of hope amidst the darkness.

Throughout the chapters of this cookbook, I endeavor to demystify the complexities of osteoporosis, providing you with a comprehensive understanding of this condition and the steps you can take to mitigate its impact on your life. From the basics of bone health to practical tips for incorporating nutrient-rich foods into your diet, each section is designed to equip you with the knowledge and tools you need to thrive.

But beyond mere information lies a deeper truth—a truth that speaks to the transformative power of food as medicine. As a physician, I have long recognized the pivotal role that nutrition plays in promoting health and healing. In the case of osteoporosis, a well-balanced diet can serve as a cornerstone of management, providing essential nutrients that support bone strength and density.

With this in mind, I have curated a selection of recipes that not only tantalize the taste buds but also nourish the body from within. From vibrant salads to hearty soups, from satisfying main courses to wholesome snacks, each dish is thoughtfully crafted to deliver a potent dose of bone-boosting nutrients. Drawing inspiration from a diverse array of culinary traditions, these recipes celebrate the rich tapestry of flavors and ingredients that make eating a joyous and rewarding experience.

As you explore these recipes, I encourage you to approach each meal with mindfulness and intention, savoring not only the flavors but also the nourishment it provides. Embrace the ritual of cooking as an act of self-care—a gift you give yourself each day, imbued with love and compassion. And remember, the journey to optimal health is not a sprint but a marathon—a steady progression towards wellness that is as much about balance and moderation as it is about dedication and perseverance.

In closing, I extend my deepest gratitude to you, dear reader, for entrusting me with your health and well-being. It is my sincere hope that this cookbook serves as a guiding light on your path to better bone health—a source of inspiration, empowerment, and joy.

With warmest regards,

Dr. Samantha Hayes

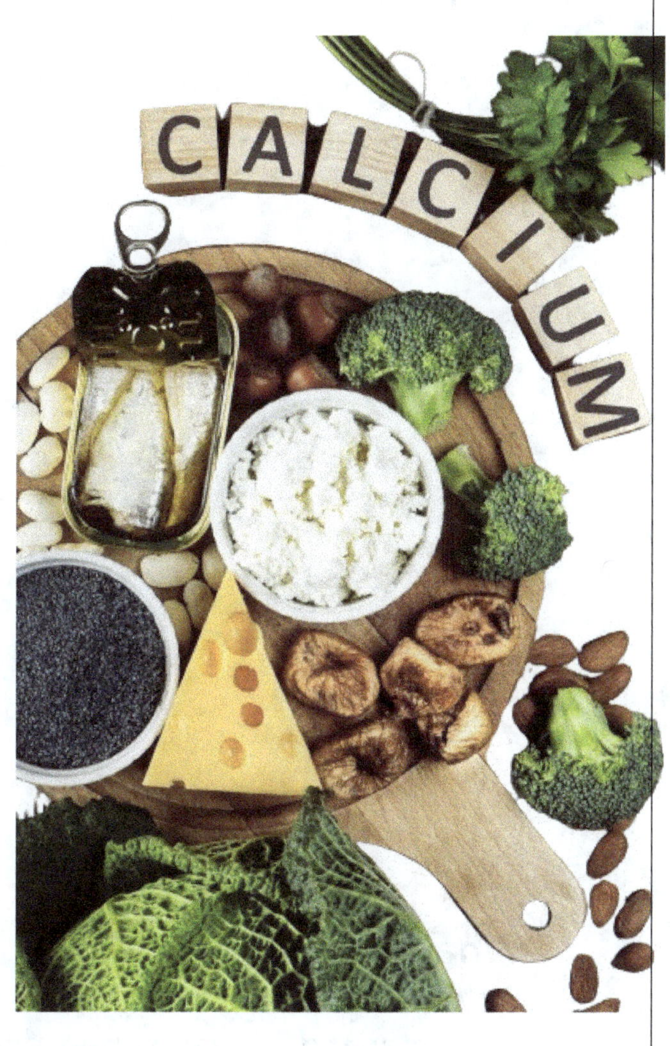
CALCIUM

CHAPTER 1

Understanding Osteoporosis

What is Osteoporosis?

Osteoporosis is a medical condition characterized by weakened and porous bones, making them more prone to fractures. The word "osteoporosis" itself translates to "porous bones," reflecting the fundamental issue at the heart of this condition.

Our bones are dynamic structures, constantly being broken down and rebuilt in a process known as bone remodeling. In a healthy individual, this remodeling process is balanced, with new bone formation keeping pace with old bone removal. However, in osteoporosis, this balance is disrupted, resulting in a net loss of bone density and strength over time.

Several factors contribute to the development of osteoporosis, including age, genetics, hormonal changes (particularly in women during menopause), certain medical conditions, and lifestyle factors such as diet, physical activity, and smoking.

One of the most concerning aspects of osteoporosis is its silent progression. Often, individuals may not be aware they have osteoporosis until they experience a fracture, typically in the spine, hip, or wrist. These fractures can have significant consequences, leading to pain, disability, loss of independence, and in severe cases, even mortality.

Diagnosis of osteoporosis is typically made through bone density testing, such as a Dual-energy X-ray Absorptiometry (DXA) scan. This test measures bone mineral density (BMD) and compares it to the BMD of a healthy young adult, providing a T-score that indicates the relative strength of the bones.

Treatment and management of osteoporosis focus on preventing fractures and preserving bone health. This often involves a multifaceted approach, including lifestyle modifications (such as a balanced diet rich in calcium and vitamin D, regular weight-bearing exercise, and avoidance of smoking and excessive alcohol consumption), medication to slow bone loss or stimulate bone formation, and fall prevention strategies.

In summary, osteoporosis is a condition characterized by weakened and porous bones, resulting from an imbalance in the bone remodeling process. It is a silent but serious condition that increases the risk of fractures and can have significant impacts on an individual's health and quality of life. Early detection, prevention, and management are crucial in mitigating the effects of osteoporosis and preserving bone health.

Types of Osteoporosis

Osteoporosis, often referred to as the "silent disease," is a condition characterized by weakened and brittle bones, making them more susceptible to fractures. While osteoporosis itself manifests similarly across different individuals, it can be categorized into several types based on underlying causes or specific characteristics. Understanding these types is crucial for accurate diagnosis and effective management of the condition. Here are some common types of osteoporosis:

Primary Osteoporosis

- ✓ **Postmenopausal Osteoporosis:** This is the most common type of osteoporosis and typically occurs in women after menopause due to a decline in estrogen levels, which accelerates bone loss.

- ✓ **Age-Related Osteoporosis:** As people age, bone density naturally decreases, increasing the risk of osteoporosis. This type is more prevalent in both men and women as they advance in age.

Secondary Osteoporosis

Secondary osteoporosis results from underlying medical conditions or medications that affect bone health. Examples include:

- Endocrine disorders such as hyperthyroidism, hyperparathyroidism, and Cushing's syndrome.

- Gastrointestinal disorders like celiac disease, inflammatory bowel disease, or gastric bypass surgery.

- Chronic conditions such as rheumatoid arthritis, chronic kidney disease, or HIV/AIDS.

- Prolonged use of corticosteroids, certain anticonvulsants, or chemotherapy.

Idiopathic Juvenile Osteoporosis

This rare type of osteoporosis affects children and adolescents, leading to reduced bone density and an increased risk of fractures. The exact cause is unknown, hence the term "idiopathic."

Localized Osteoporosis

Unlike generalized osteoporosis that affects the entire skeleton, localized osteoporosis occurs in specific regions of the body, often due to immobilization or disuse. For example, after a prolonged period of casting or immobilization following a fracture, the bones within the immobilized limb may experience localized bone loss.

Secondary to Medications

Certain medications, particularly long-term use of corticosteroids (glucocorticoids), can induce osteoporosis by interfering with bone remodeling and calcium absorption, leading to decreased bone density and increased fracture risk.

High Turnover Osteoporosis

In some cases, bone turnover is increased, resulting in a condition known as high-turnover osteoporosis. This can occur in conditions such as hyperparathyroidism or Paget's disease of bone.

Causes of Osteoporosis

Osteoporosis is a multifactorial condition influenced by various genetic, hormonal, lifestyle, and medical factors. Understanding the underlying causes of osteoporosis is crucial for effective prevention and management. Here are some of the primary causes:

Aging: One of the most significant risk factors for osteoporosis is aging. As people age, bone density naturally decreases, and bone turnover slows down, making bones more susceptible to fractures.

Hormonal Changes

- **Estrogen Deficiency:** In women, estrogen plays a crucial role in maintaining bone density. After menopause, estrogen levels decline, leading to accelerated bone loss and an increased risk of osteoporosis.

- **Testosterone Deficiency:** Low testosterone levels in men, particularly due to aging or certain medical conditions, can also contribute to bone loss and osteoporosis.

Genetics: Family history and genetics play a significant role in determining an individual's risk of osteoporosis. People with a family history of osteoporosis or a family history of fractures may be at higher risk.

Nutritional Deficiencies: Inadequate intake of calcium, vitamin D, and other essential nutrients necessary for bone health can contribute to the development of osteoporosis. Calcium is a key building block of bone tissue, and vitamin D helps the body absorb calcium efficiently.

Lifestyle Factors

- **Sedentary Lifestyle:** Lack of weight-bearing exercise and physical activity can weaken bones and contribute to bone loss.

- **Smoking:** Smoking has been linked to decreased bone density and an increased risk of fractures.

- **Excessive Alcohol Consumption:** Heavy alcohol consumption can interfere with the body's ability to absorb calcium and negatively impact bone health.

Medical Conditions

- **Endocrine Disorders:** Conditions such as hyperthyroidism, hyperparathyroidism, Cushing's syndrome, and diabetes can affect bone metabolism and increase the risk of osteoporosis.

- **Gastrointestinal Disorders:** Conditions like celiac disease, inflammatory bowel disease, and gastric bypass surgery can impair nutrient absorption and lead to osteoporosis.

- **Rheumatologic Disorders:** Rheumatoid arthritis and other autoimmune conditions can cause inflammation and bone damage, contributing to osteoporosis.

- **Chronic Kidney Disease:** Kidney dysfunction can disrupt calcium and vitamin D metabolism, leading to bone loss and osteoporosis.

Medications
- **Corticosteroids:** Long-term use of corticosteroid medications, such

as prednisone, can lead to bone loss and osteoporosis.

- **Certain Medications:** Some other medications, including certain anticonvulsants, proton pump inhibitors (PPIs), and cancer treatments, may also increase the risk of osteoporosis.

Low Body Weight or BMI: Being underweight or having a low body mass index (BMI) can increase the risk of osteoporosis, as there may be less bone mass to begin with.

Symptoms of Osteoporosis

Osteoporosis is often referred to as a "silent disease" because it typically progresses without noticeable symptoms until a fracture occurs. However, there are some signs and symptoms associated with osteoporosis that may indicate bone loss or an increased risk of fractures. Here are the key symptoms to be aware of:

Height Loss: Osteoporosis-related fractures, particularly in the vertebrae of the spine, can lead to a loss of height over time. This height loss may be gradual and progressive.

Back Pain: Compression fractures in the spine can cause persistent or worsening back pain. This pain may be localized to the affected area and may worsen with movement, standing, or lifting.

Bone Fractures: Osteoporosis weakens bones, increasing the risk of fractures, especially in the hip, spine (vertebrae), and wrist. Fractures may occur with minimal trauma or from activities of daily living, such as lifting, bending, or falling from standing height.

Stooped Posture: Compression fractures in the spine can lead to a forward curvature of the upper back (kyphosis) and a stooped posture. This change in posture may be more noticeable over time and can contribute to height loss and back pain.

Decreased Grip Strength: Weakening of the bones in the hands and wrists due to osteoporosis may lead to a decrease in grip strength, making it more challenging to perform tasks that require hand strength.

Brittle Nails: In some cases, osteoporosis may manifest with changes in nail health, including increased brittleness or susceptibility to breakage.

Tooth Loss: Severe osteoporosis may affect the bones of the jaw, leading to tooth loss or other dental issues.

It's important to note that while these symptoms may indicate the presence of osteoporosis, they can also be caused by other conditions. Additionally, not all individuals with osteoporosis experience symptoms, especially in the early stages of the disease.

If you experience any of these symptoms or have concerns about your bone health, it's essential to consult with a healthcare professional. Early detection, diagnosis, and management of osteoporosis can help prevent fractures and reduce the risk of complications associated with this condition. Regular bone density testing and evaluation of fracture risk factors are recommended, especially for individuals at higher risk due to age, gender, family history, or other medical conditions.

Preventive Measures for Osteoporosis

Preventive measures play a crucial role in reducing the risk of osteoporosis and maintaining bone health throughout life.

Nutritious Diet

- **Ensure an adequate intake of calcium:** Calcium is essential for building and maintaining strong bones. Good dietary sources of calcium include dairy products, leafy green vegetables, tofu, almonds, and fortified foods.

- **Get enough vitamin D**: Vitamin D is necessary for calcium absorption and bone health. Spend time outdoors in sunlight, consume vitamin D-rich foods such as fatty fish, egg yolks, and fortified foods, or consider taking a vitamin D supplement if recommended by a healthcare professional.

- **Maintain a balanced diet:** Eating a variety of nutrient-rich foods, including fruits, vegetables, whole grains, lean proteins, and healthy fats, provides the body with essential vitamins and minerals needed for optimal bone health.

Regular Exercise

- **Engage in weight-bearing and muscle-strengthening exercises:** Weight-bearing exercises, such as walking, jogging, dancing, and strength training, help stimulate bone growth and maintain bone density. Aim for at least 30 minutes of moderate-intensity exercise most days of the week.

- **Include balance and flexibility exercises:** Activities like yoga, tai chi, and Pilates can improve balance, coordination, and flexibility, reducing the risk of falls and fractures.

- **Avoid sedentary behavior:** Limiting prolonged sitting or lying down can help maintain bone strength and overall health. Incorporate regular physical activity into your daily routine.

Lifestyle modifications

  - **Avoid smoking:** Smoking has been linked to decreased bone density and an increased risk of fractures. If you smoke, consider quitting or seeking support to quit smoking.

- **Limit alcohol consumption:** Excessive alcohol intake can interfere with calcium absorption and bone health. Aim to drink alcohol in moderation, if at all, following recommended guidelines.

Bone Health Screening

Discuss bone density testing with a healthcare professional: Bone density testing, such as a Dual-energy X-ray Absorptiometry (DXA) scan, can assess bone density and fracture risk. Talk to your healthcare provider about when and how often you should be screened based on your age, gender, risk factors, and medical history.

Medication Management

If necessary, follow prescribed medications: In some cases, healthcare providers may recommend medications to prevent or treat osteoporosis, particularly for individuals at higher risk or those with low bone density. Adhere to prescribed medication regimens and discuss any concerns or side effects with a healthcare professional.

Fall Prevention
Take steps to prevent falls: Reduce the risk of falls by ensuring adequate lighting, removing hazards, using assistive devices if needed, wearing proper footwear, and participating in balance and strength training exercises.

Chapter 2
Importance of Nutrition in Managing Osteoporosis

Nutrition plays a fundamental role in managing osteoporosis, a condition characterized by weakened and porous bones. The right balance of nutrients supports bone health by providing essential building blocks for bone formation, maintaining bone density, and reducing the risk of fractures. Here's why nutrition is crucial in managing osteoporosis:

Calcium and Vitamin D Absorption

Calcium is a primary mineral essential for bone health, as it contributes to bone density and strength. However, calcium absorption is dependent on adequate levels of vitamin D. Vitamin D helps the body absorb calcium from the diet and regulates calcium metabolism. Adequate intake of both calcium and vitamin D is critical for maintaining optimal bone health and reducing the risk of osteoporosis-related fractures.

Bone Formation and Remodeling

Nutrients such as calcium, phosphorus, magnesium, and vitamin K are involved in bone formation and remodeling processes. These nutrients contribute to the production of bone matrix and the mineralization of bone tissue, helping to maintain bone strength and integrity. Inadequate intake of these nutrients can impair bone formation and increase the risk of bone loss, leading to osteoporosis.

Prevention of Bone Loss
Certain nutrients, such as calcium, vitamin D, and protein, play a role in preventing bone loss associated with aging and other risk factors. Consuming sufficient amounts of these nutrients through diet or supplementation can help preserve bone density and reduce the risk of fractures.

Additionally, antioxidants and anti-inflammatory nutrients found in fruits, vegetables, and whole grains may help protect bone health by reducing oxidative stress and inflammation, which can contribute to bone loss.

Muscle Strength and Balance

Nutrition also influences muscle health, which is important for maintaining balance, stability, and mobility, thus reducing the risk of falls and fractures.

Adequate protein intake is essential for muscle maintenance and repair, while vitamin D plays a role in muscle function and coordination. Consuming a balanced diet that includes protein-rich foods and vitamin D-rich sources can support muscle strength and reduce the risk of falls.

Overall Health and Wellbeing

A nutritious diet supports overall health and well-being, which indirectly contributes to bone health. Eating a variety of nutrient-rich foods provides essential vitamins, minerals, antioxidants, and phytonutrients that support immune function, reduce inflammation, and promote overall health.

Maintaining a healthy body weight through proper nutrition and regular physical activity can also help reduce the risk of osteoporosis and improve outcomes for individuals with the condition.

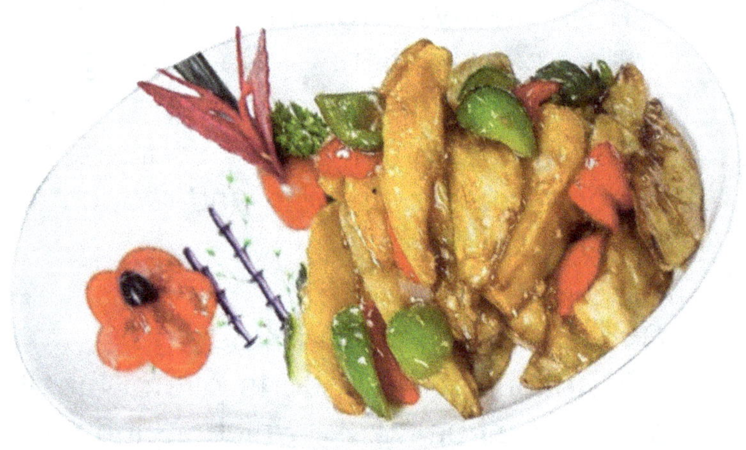

Foods to Eat for Stronger Bones

Building Stronger bones begins with a balanced diet rich in nutrients essential for bone health. Here's a list of foods that are beneficial for strengthening bones

Dairy Products: Milk, Yogurt, Cheese (such as cheddar, mozzarella, and Swiss)

Leafy Green Vegetables: Kale, Spinach, Collard greens

Calcium-Fortified Foods: Fortified plant-based milk (almond, soy, coconut), Fortified orange juice, Fortified cereals

Fatty Fish: Salmon, Sardines, Mackerel

Tofu and Soy Products: Firm tofu, Tempeh, Edamame

Nuts and Seeds: Almonds, Chia seeds, Sesame seeds

Beans and Legumes: Chickpeas (garbanzo beans), Black beans, Lentils

Whole Grains: Oats, Quinoa, Brown rice

Eggs: Whole eggs, Egg yolks

Lean Protein Sources: Chicken breast, Turkey, Lean beef

Berries: Strawberries, Blueberries, Raspberries

Cruciferous Vegetables: Broccoli, Brussels sprouts, Cauliflower

Sweet Potatoes: Rich in vitamin A, which supports bone growth and development.

Fortified Margarine or Spreads: Some spreads are fortified with vitamin D, which aids in calcium absorption.

Fortified Plant-Based Milk Alternatives: Fortified almond milk, soy milk, or coconut milk can provide calcium and vitamin D.

Seaweed: Particularly kelp, which is high in calcium and magnesium.

Prunes: Prunes contain vitamin K and antioxidants that support bone health.

Bell Peppers: Red, yellow, and orange bell peppers are high in vitamin C, which is important for collagen production in bones.

Lean Meats: Such as skinless poultry and lean cuts of beef or pork, which provide protein and other nutrients necessary for bone health.

Foods to Avoid to Reduce Bone Loss

Carbonated Beverages: Regular consumption of soda has been linked to decreased bone density.

Excessive Alcohol: Heavy alcohol consumption can interfere with calcium absorption and increase the risk of fractures.

Salty Foods: High-sodium diets can lead to calcium loss through urine and may weaken bones over time.

Processed Foods: Highly processed foods often lack essential nutrients and may contribute to poor bone health.

High-Caffeine Beverages: Excessive caffeine intake can interfere with calcium absorption and may increase the risk of bone loss.

Excessive Red Meat: While lean cuts of red meat can be part of a balanced diet, excessive consumption may have negative effects on bone health.

Foods High in Oxalates: Some foods high in oxalates, such as spinach and rhubarb, can bind to calcium and reduce its absorption.

High-Phosphorus Foods: Foods high in phosphorus, such as soda and processed meats, may interfere with calcium balance in the body.

Sugary Snacks and Desserts: Diets high in added sugars have been associated with decreased bone density and increased fracture risk.

Excessive Sodium: High-sodium diets can lead to increased calcium excretion in the urine and may contribute to bone loss over time.

Fried Foods: Foods fried in unhealthy oils may contribute to inflammation and oxidative stress, which can affect bone health.

High-Sugar Breakfast Cereals: Some breakfast cereals are high in added sugars and may lack essential nutrients necessary for bone health.

Refined Carbohydrates: Diets high in refined carbohydrates may be low in essential nutrients and may not support optimal bone health.

Processed Meats: Processed meats, such as bacon, sausage, and deli meats, are often high in sodium and may contain preservatives that can affect bone health.

Alcohol: Excessive alcohol consumption can interfere with calcium absorption and increase the risk of fractures.

Excessive Caffeine: High caffeine intake can lead to increased calcium excretion in the urine and may negatively affect bone health.

High-Sodium Foods: Diets high in sodium can lead to increased calcium excretion in the urine and may contribute to bone loss over time.

Sugary Drinks: Regular consumption of sugary drinks has been associated with decreased bone density and increased fracture risk.

Refined Grains: Diets high in refined grains may lack essential nutrients necessary for bone health and may not support optimal bone density.

High-Sodium Condiments: Condiments such as soy sauce, barbecue sauce, and salad dressings can be high in sodium and may contribute to bone loss when consumed in excess.

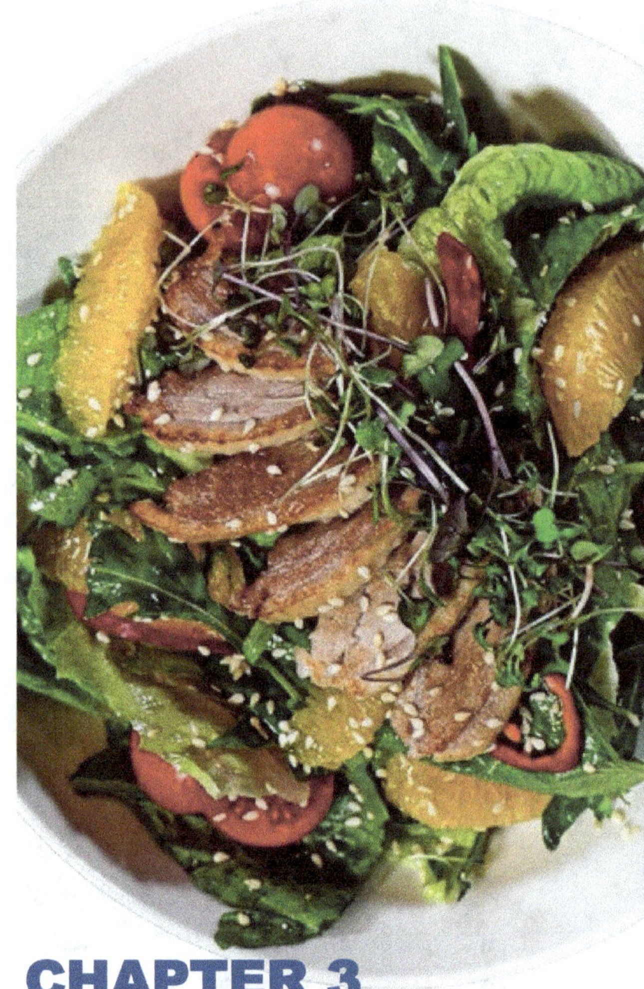

CHAPTER 3
Osteoporosis Diet Recipes
Breakfast Recipes

1. Calcium-Rich Smoothie
Ingredients:

1 cup spinach
1/2 cup kale
1 ripe banana
1/2 cup Greek yogurt (plain or vanilla, fortified with vitamin D and calcium)
1/2 cup almond milk (fortified with calcium)
1 tablespoon chia seeds
1/4 cup strawberries, sliced
Ice cubes (optional)

Instructions:
In a blender, combine spinach, kale, banana, Greek yogurt, almond milk, and chia seeds.
Blend until smooth and creamy.
Add sliced strawberries and ice cubes if desired, and blend again until well combined.
Pour into glasses and serve immediately.

Nutritional Value (per serving)
Calories: 220 kcal
Protein: 12g
Fat: 6g
Carbohydrates: 35g

Fiber: 9g
Calcium: 30% DV
Vitamin D: 25% DV

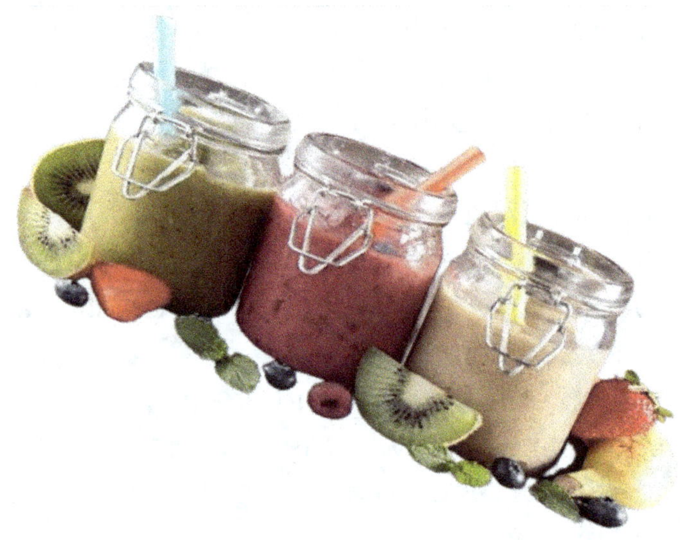

2. Greek Yogurt Parfait with Berries and Almonds

Ingredients:

1 cup Greek yogurt (plain or vanilla, fortified with calcium and vitamin D)
1/4 cup granola (low-sugar)

1/4 cup mixed berries (such as strawberries, blueberries, raspberries)
1 tablespoon almonds, sliced
1 teaspoon honey (optional)

Instructions:

In a serving glass or bowl, layer Greek yogurt, granola, mixed berries, and sliced almonds.
Repeat the layers until ingredients are used up.
Drizzle with honey if desired.
Serve immediately or refrigerate until ready to eat.

Nutritional Value (per serving)

Calories: 280 kcal
Protein: 18g
Fat: 10g
Carbohydrates: 30g
Fiber: 5g
Calcium: 20% DV
Vitamin D: 15% DV

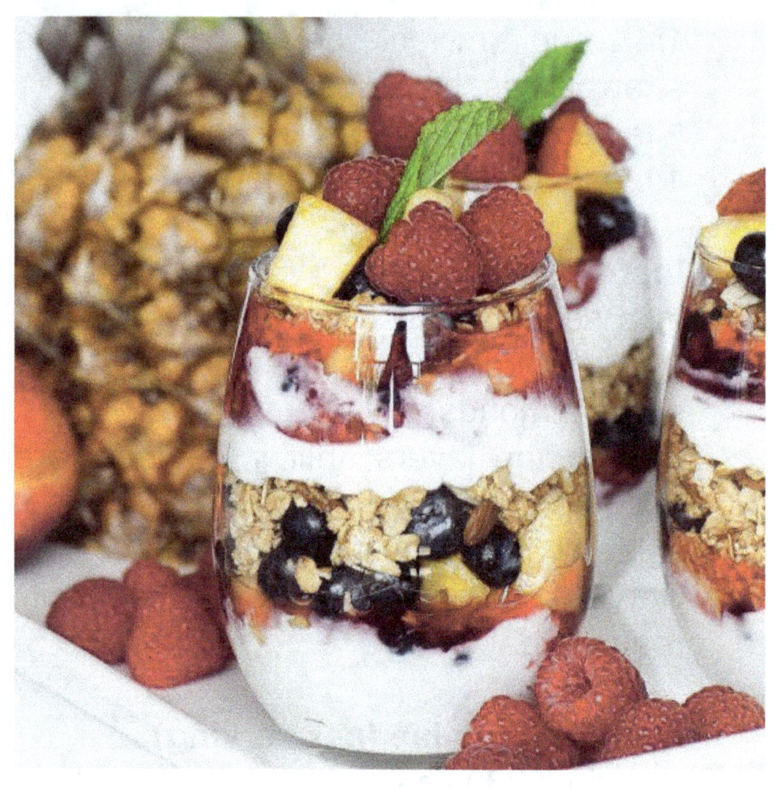

3.   Spinach   and   Mushroom Frittata

Ingredients:
4 large eggs
1 cup fresh spinach, chopped
1/2 cup mushrooms, sliced
1/4 cup red bell pepper, diced
1/4 cup onion, diced

1/4 cup low-fat cheese (such as feta or mozzarella)
1 tablespoon olive oil
Salt and pepper to taste

Instructions:

Preheat the oven to 350°F (175°C).

In a mixing bowl, whisk together eggs, salt, and pepper.

Heat olive oil in an oven-safe skillet over medium heat. Add onions and bell peppers, and sauté until softened.

Add mushrooms and spinach to the skillet and cook until spinach is wilted and mushrooms are tender.

Pour the whisked eggs evenly over the vegetables in the skillet.

Sprinkle cheese on top and cook for a few minutes until the edges begin to set.

Transfer the skillet to the preheated oven and bake for 12-15 minutes until the frittata is set and lightly golden on top.

Remove from the oven, slice into wedges, and serve hot.

Nutritional Value (per serving)

Calories: 220 kcal
Protein: 14g
Fat: 15g
Carbohydrates: 7g
Fiber: 2g
Calcium: 10% DV
Vitamin D: 8% DV

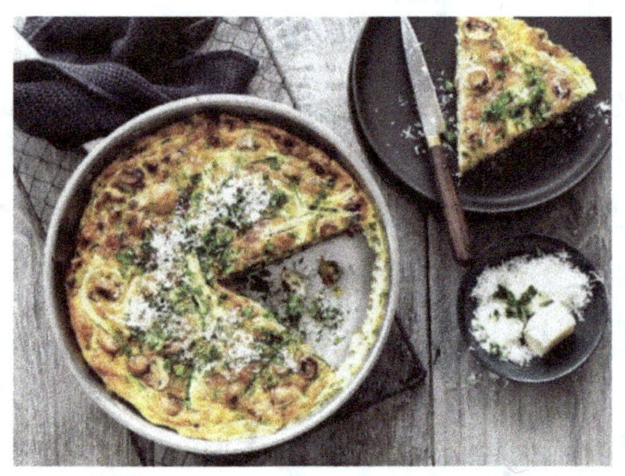

4. Avocado Toast with Poached Egg

Ingredients:

2 slices whole grain bread
1 ripe avocado, mashed
2 large eggs
1 tablespoon white vinegar
Salt and pepper to taste
Red pepper flakes (optional)

Instructions:

Toast the whole grain bread slices until golden brown.

Spread mashed avocado evenly on each slice of toast.

In a saucepan, bring water to a gentle simmer. Add white vinegar.

Crack one egg into a small bowl. Using a spoon, create a whirlpool in the simmering water and carefully slide the egg into the center of the whirlpool. Repeat with the second egg.

Poach the eggs for about 3-4 minutes until the whites are set but the yolks are still runny.

Using a slotted spoon, remove the poached eggs from the water and place them on top of the avocado toast.

Season with salt, pepper, and red pepper flakes if desired.

Serve immediately.

Nutritional Value (per serving)

Calories: 320 kcal

Protein: 15g

Fat: 20g

Carbohydrates: 25g
Fiber: 10g
Calcium: 8% DV
Vitamin D: 6% DV

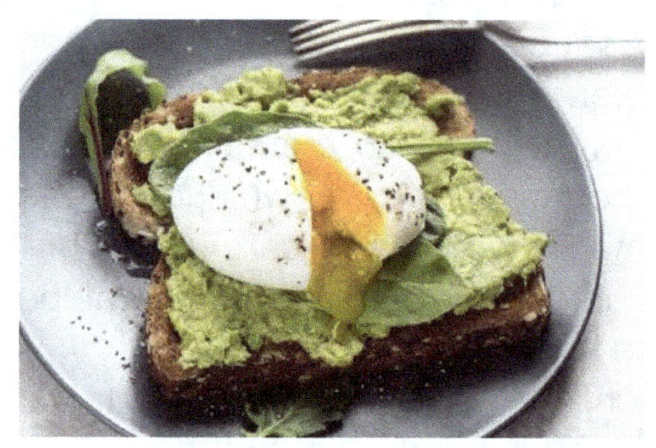

5. Whole Grain Pancakes With Blueberries And Walnuts

Ingredients:
1 cup whole wheat flour
1 tablespoon baking powder
1 tablespoon honey or maple syrup
1 cup almond milk (fortified with calcium)
1 large egg
1 teaspoon vanilla extract

1/2 cup blueberries
1/4 cup walnuts, chopped
Cooking spray or butter for greasing the skillet

Instructions:

In a mixing bowl, whisk together whole wheat flour and baking powder.
In another bowl, whisk together honey or maple syrup, almond milk, egg, and vanilla extract until well combined.
Pour the wet ingredients into the dry ingredients and stir until just combined. Be careful not to overmix.
Heat a skillet or griddle over medium heat and lightly grease with cooking spray or butter.
Pour 1/4 cup of batter onto the skillet for each pancake.
Sprinkle a few blueberries and chopped walnuts onto each pancake.
Cook until bubbles form on the surface of the pancakes, then flip and cook until golden brown on both sides.
Repeat with the remaining batter.

Serve warm with additional blueberries, walnuts, and a drizzle of honey or maple syrup if desired.

Nutritional Value (per serving, 2 pancakes)
Calories: 300 kcal
Protein: 10g
Fat: 10g
Carbohydrates: 45g
Fiber: 6g
Calcium: 15% DV
Vitamin D: 10% DV

6. Spinach and Feta Breakfast Wrap
Ingredients:
2 large whole grain tortillas
4 large eggs, scrambled
1 cup fresh spinach leaves
1/4 cup crumbled feta cheese
1/4 cup diced tomatoes
2 tablespoons salsa or hot sauce (optional)

Salt and pepper to taste

Instructions:
Heat a non-stick skillet over medium heat.
Add scrambled eggs to the skillet and cook until set.
Warm the tortillas in a separate skillet or microwave until soft and pliable.
Divide the scrambled eggs evenly between the two tortillas.
Top each tortilla with fresh spinach leaves, crumbled feta cheese, diced tomatoes, and salsa or hot sauce if desired.
Season with salt and pepper to taste.
Roll up the tortillas, tucking in the sides to enclose the filling.
Slice in half and serve warm.

Nutritional Value (per serving)
Calories: 280 kcal   Calcium: 15% DV
Protein: 20g   Vitamin D: 10% DV
Fat: 15g
Carbohydrates: 20g

Fiber: 5g

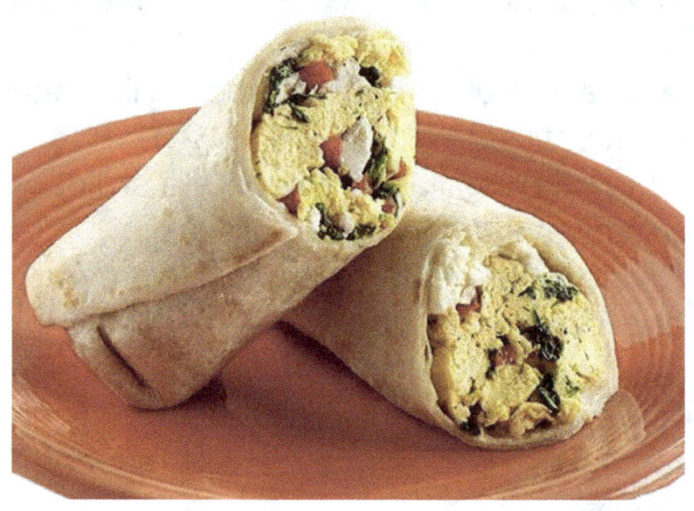

7. Overnight Oats with Almond Butter and Banana
Ingredients:
1/2 cup rolled oats
1/2 cup almond milk (fortified with calcium)
1 tablespoon almond butter
1/2 ripe banana, mashed
1 tablespoon chia seeds

1 teaspoon honey or maple syrup (optional)
Sliced almonds for topping

Instructions:

In a mason jar or airtight container, combine rolled oats, almond milk, almond butter, mashed banana, chia seeds, and honey or maple syrup if using.

Stir well to combine all ingredients.

Cover the jar or container and refrigerate overnight, or for at least 4 hours, to allow the oats to soften and absorb the liquid.

Before serving, give the oats a good stir and add a splash of almond milk if needed to reach your desired consistency.

Top with sliced almonds before serving.

Nutritional Value (per serving)

Calories: 320 kcal   Calcium: 20% DV

Protein: 10g   Vitamin D: 15% DV

Fat: 12g

Carbohydrates: 45g
Fiber: 8g

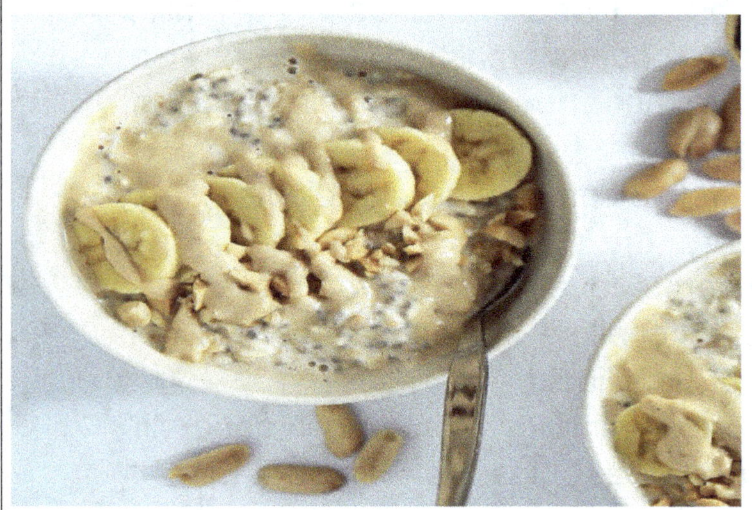

8. Veggie Breakfast Burrito
Ingredients:
2 large whole grain tortillas
4 large eggs, scrambled
1/2 cup black beans, drained and rinsed

1/4 cup shredded cheddar cheese
1/4 cup salsa
1/4 cup diced bell peppers
1/4 cup diced onions
Salt and pepper to taste

Instructions:
Heat a non-stick skillet over medium heat.
Add scrambled eggs, black beans, diced bell peppers, and diced onions to the skillet.
Cook until eggs are set and vegetables are tender.
Warm the tortillas in a separate skillet or microwave until soft and pliable.
Divide the egg and vegetable mixture evenly between the two tortillas.
Top each tortilla with shredded cheddar cheese and salsa.
Season with salt and pepper to taste.
Roll up the tortillas, tucking in the sides to enclose the filling.
Slice in half and serve warm.

Nutritional Value (per serving)
Calories: 350 kcal

Protein: 20g
Fat: 15g
Carbohydrates: 35g
Fiber: 8g
Calcium: 15% DV
Vitamin D: 10% DV

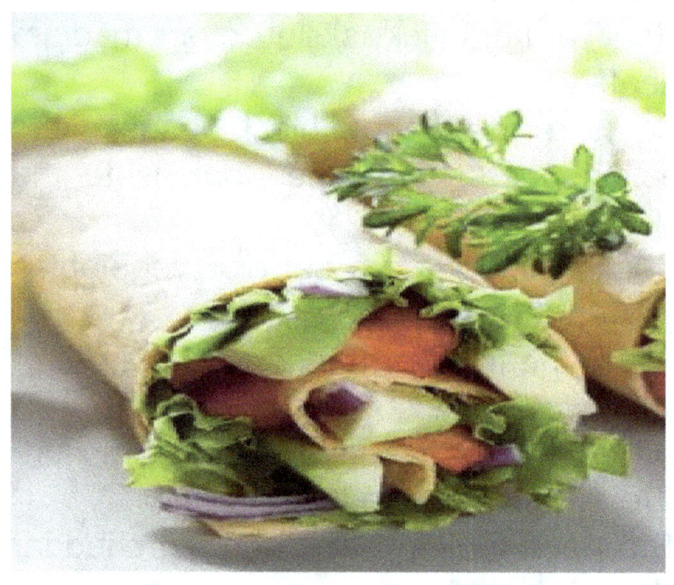

9. Cottage Cheese and Fruit Bowl Ingredients:

1/2 cup low-fat cottage cheese
1/2 cup mixed berries (such as strawberries, blueberries, raspberries)
1/4 cup sliced kiwi

1 tablespoon chopped nuts (such as almonds, walnuts, or pecans)
1 teaspoon honey (optional)

Instructions:
Spoon cottage cheese into a serving bowl.
Top with mixed berries, sliced kiwi, and chopped nuts.
Drizzle with honey if desired.
Serve immediately.

Nutritional Value (per serving)
Calories: 250 kcal
Protein: 20g
Fat: 10g
Carbohydrates: 20g
Fiber: 5g
Calcium: 15% DV
Vitamin D: 10% DV

10. Quinoa Breakfast Bowl
Ingredients:
1/2 cup cooked quinoa
1/2 cup Greek yogurt (plain or vanilla, fortified with calcium and vitamin D)

1/4 cup mixed berries (such as strawberries, blueberries, raspberries)
1 tablespoon sliced almonds
1 teaspoon honey or maple syrup (optional)

Instructions:
In a serving bowl, layer cooked quinoa and Greek yogurt.
Top with mixed berries and sliced almonds.
Drizzle with honey or maple syrup if desired.
Serve immediately.

Nutritional Value (per serving)
Calories: 280 kcal   Vitamin D: 15% DV
Protein: 20g
Fat: 8g   Fiber: 5g
Carbohydrates: 35g
Calcium: 20% DV

Lunch Recipes

1. Grilled Salmon Salad
Ingredients:
4 oz grilled salmon fillet

2 cups mixed greens (spinach, kale, arugula)
1/4 cup cherry tomatoes, halved
1/4 cup cucumber, sliced
1/4 avocado, sliced
1 tablespoon olive oil
1 tablespoon balsamic vinegar
Salt and pepper to taste

Instructions:

Season the salmon fillet with salt and pepper and grill until cooked through.
In a large bowl, toss mixed greens, cherry tomatoes, cucumber, and avocado slices.
Drizzle olive oil and balsamic vinegar over the salad and toss to coat.
Place the grilled salmon on top of the salad.
Serve immediately.

Nutritional Value (per serving)

Calories: 350 kcal
Protein: 25g
Fat: 22g
Carbohydrates: 15g

Fiber: 6g
Calcium: 8% DV
Vitamin D: 15% DV

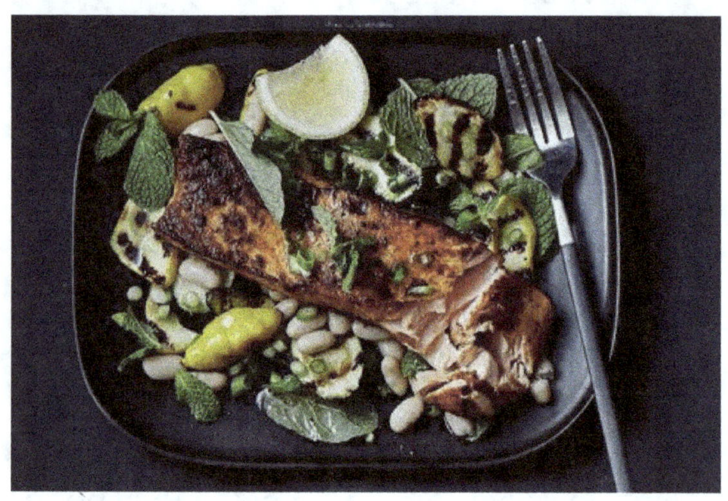

2. Quinoa Stuffed Bell peppers
Ingredients:
2 large bell peppers, halved and seeds removed
1 cup cooked quinoa

1/2 cup black beans, drained and rinsed
1/4 cup corn kernels
1/4 cup diced tomatoes
1/4 cup diced red onion
1/4 cup shredded cheddar cheese
1 tablespoon olive oil
1 teaspoon chili powder
Salt and pepper to taste

Instructions:

Preheat the oven to 375°F (190°C).

In a large bowl, mix cooked quinoa, black beans, corn kernels, diced tomatoes, diced red onion, shredded cheddar cheese, olive oil, chili powder, salt, and pepper.

Stuff each bell pepper half with the quinoa mixture.

Place the stuffed bell peppers on a baking sheet lined with parchment paper.

Bake for 25-30 minutes until the peppers are tender and the filling is heated through.

Serve hot.

Nutritional Value (per serving, 1 stuffed pepper half)
Calories: 200 kcal
Protein: 8g
Fat: 8g
Carbohydrates: 25g
Fiber: 5g
Calcium: 10% DV
Vitamin D: 6% DV

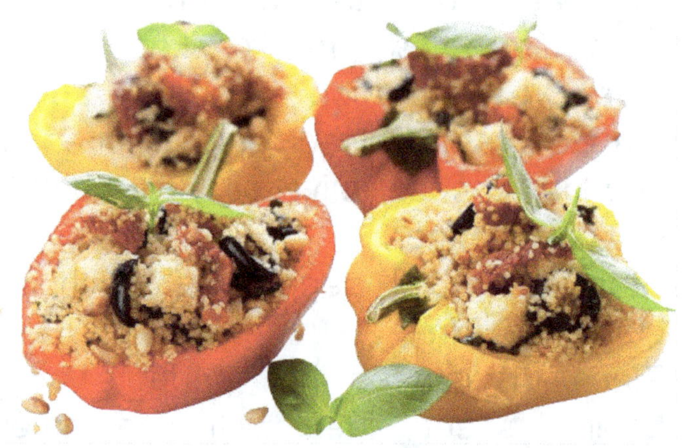

3. Chicken and Vegetable Stir-Fry

Ingredients:
4 oz boneless, skinless chicken breast, sliced

1 cup broccoli florets
1/2 cup bell peppers, sliced
1/2 cup snap peas
1/4 cup carrots, sliced
2 tablespoons low-sodium soy sauce
1 tablespoon olive oil
1 teaspoon minced garlic
1/2 teaspoon grated ginger
Sesame seeds for garnish (optional)
Cooked brown rice for serving

Instructions:

Heat olive oil in a large skillet or wok over medium-high heat.

Add minced garlic and grated ginger to the skillet and cook for 1 minute until fragrant.

Add sliced chicken breast to the skillet and cook until browned and cooked through.

Add broccoli florets, bell peppers, snap peas, and carrots to the skillet and stir-fry until vegetables are tender-crisp.

Drizzle low-sodium soy sauce over the stir-fry and toss to coat.

Remove from heat and sprinkle with sesame seeds if desired.

Serve hot over cooked brown rice.

Nutritional Value (per serving)
Calories: 300 kcal
Protein: 25g
Fat: 10g
Carbohydrates: 25g
Fiber: 5g
Calcium: 6% DV
Vitamin D: 2% DV

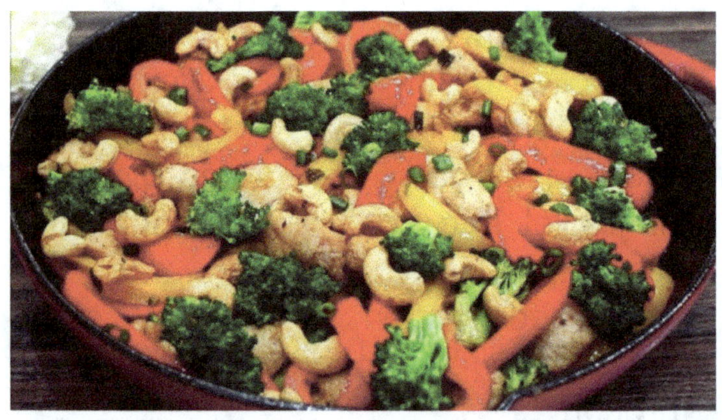

4. Lentils and Vegetable Soup
Ingredients:
1 cup dried lentils, rinsed and drained
4 cups vegetable broth
1 onion, diced
2 carrots, sliced
2 celery stalks, sliced

2 cloves garlic, minced
1 teaspoon dried thyme
1 teaspoon dried rosemary
Salt and pepper to taste
Fresh parsley for garnish

Instructions:

In a large pot, heat olive oil over medium heat.

Add diced onion, sliced carrots, and sliced celery to the pot and sauté until softened.

Add minced garlic, dried thyme, and dried rosemary to the pot and cook for 1 minute until fragrant.

Add dried lentils and vegetable broth to the pot and bring to a boil.

Reduce heat to low, cover, and simmer for 25-30 minutes until lentils are tender.

Season with salt and pepper to taste.

Ladle the soup into bowls and garnish with fresh parsley before serving.

Nutritional Value (per serving)

Calories: 250 kcal
Protein: 15g
Fat: 1g

Carbohydrates: 45g
Fiber: 15g
Calcium: 4% DV
Vitamin D: 0% DV

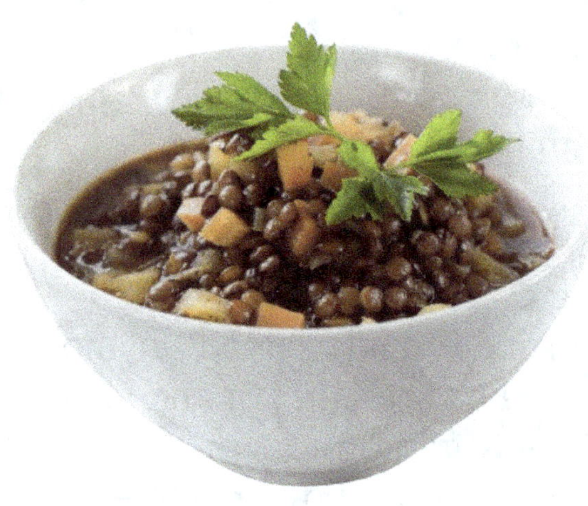

5.   Spinach   and   Mushroom Quesadilla

Ingredients:
2 large whole grain tortillas
1 cup fresh spinach leaves
1/2 cup sliced mushrooms
1/4 cup shredded mozzarella cheese
1/4 cup diced tomatoes
1/4 cup diced red onion

1 tablespoon olive oil
Salt and pepper to taste

Instructions:
Heat olive oil in a skillet over medium heat.
Add sliced mushrooms to the skillet and sauté until golden brown.
Add fresh spinach leaves to the skillet and cook until wilted.
Place one whole grain tortilla in the skillet and top with sautéed spinach and mushrooms, diced tomatoes, diced red onion, and shredded mozzarella cheese.
Place the second tortilla on top and press down gently.
Cook for 2-3 minutes on each side until golden brown and crispy.
Remove from the skillet and slice into wedges.
Serve hot with salsa or Greek yogurt for dipping.

Nutritional Value (per serving)
Calories: 300 kcal
Protein: 12g

Fat: 10g
Carbohydrates: 35g
Fiber: 5g
Calcium: 10% DV
Vitamin D: 8% DV

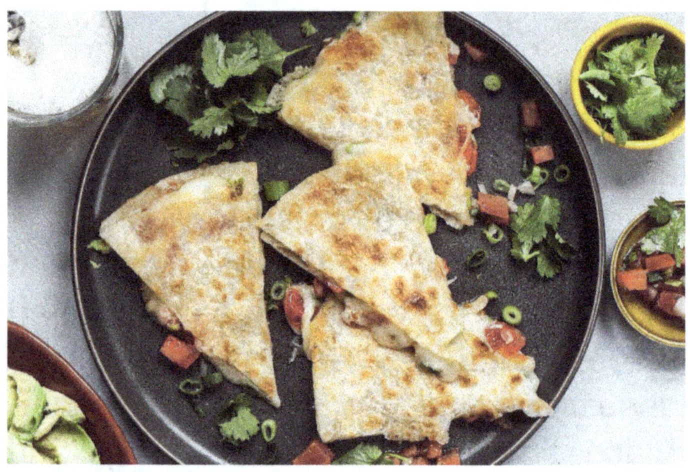

6. Turkey and Veggie Wrap
Ingredients:
1 large whole grain tortilla
3 oz sliced turkey breast
1/4 avocado, mashed
1/4 cup shredded carrots
1/4 cup sliced cucumbers
1/4 cup mixed greens (spinach, lettuce, arugula)
1 tablespoon hummus

Salt and pepper to taste

Instructions:
Lay the whole grain tortilla flat on a clean surface.
Spread mashed avocado evenly on the tortilla.
Layer sliced turkey breast, shredded carrots, sliced cucumbers, and mixed greens on top of the avocado.
Drizzle hummus over the filling and season with salt and pepper to taste.
Roll up the tortilla, tucking in the sides to enclose the filling.
Slice in half and serve immediately.

Nutritional Value (per serving)
Calories: 250 kcal
Protein: 20g
Fat: 10g
Carbohydrates: 25g
Fiber: 5g
Calcium: 8% DV
Vitamin D: 6% DV

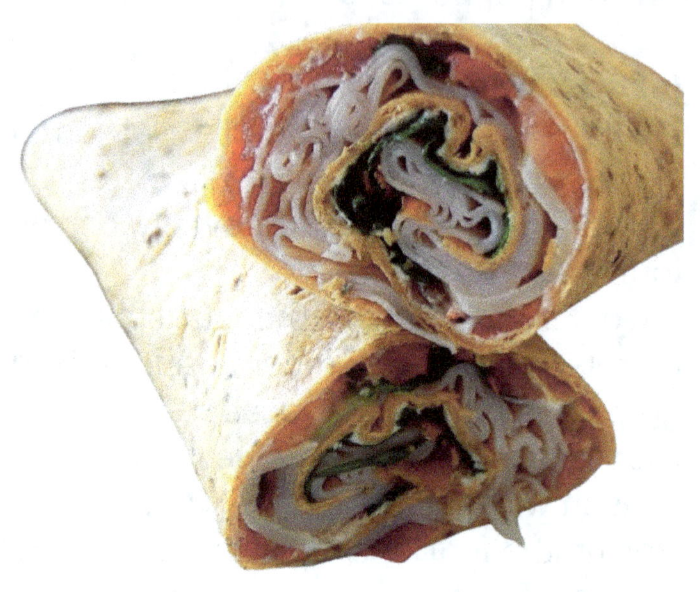

7. Chickpea Salad Sandwich
Ingredients:
1/2 cup canned chickpeas, drained and rinsed
1 tablespoon Greek yogurt
1 teaspoon Dijon mustard
1 teaspoon lemon juice
1 tablespoon chopped celery
1 tablespoon chopped red onion
Salt and pepper to taste
2 slices whole grain bread

Lettuce leaves and tomato slices for serving

Instructions:

In a mixing bowl, mash the chickpeas with a fork until slightly chunky.

Add Greek yogurt, Dijon mustard, lemon juice, chopped celery, chopped red onion, salt, and pepper to the bowl and mix until well combined.

Toast the whole grain bread slices until golden brown.

Spread the chickpea salad mixture evenly onto one slice of bread.

Top with lettuce leaves, tomato slices, and the second slice of bread.

Slice in half and serve immediately.

Nutritional Value (per serving)

Calories: 250 kcal

Protein: 10g

Fat: 5g

Carbohydrates: 40g

Fiber: 8g

Calcium: 6% DV

Vitamin D: 4% DV

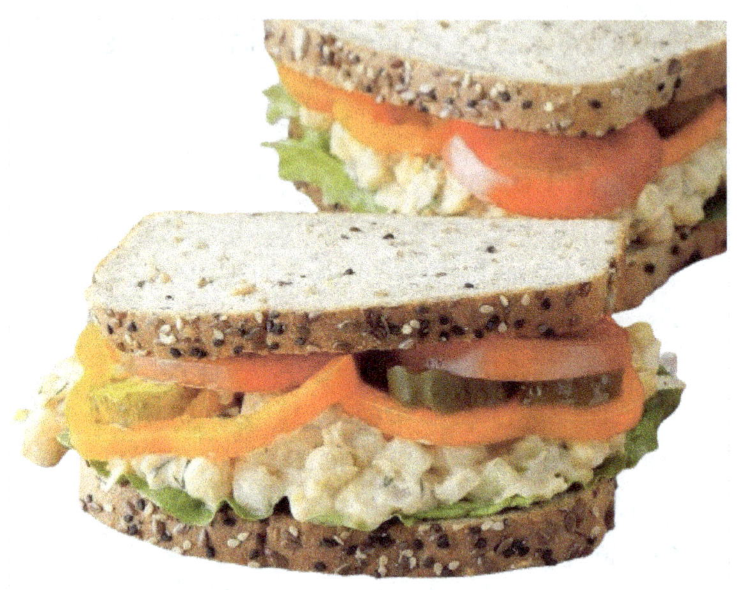

8. Spinach and Feta Turkey Burger

Ingredients:

4 oz lean ground turkey
1/4 cup fresh spinach leaves, chopped
1 tablespoon crumbled feta cheese
1/2 teaspoon minced garlic
Salt and pepper to taste
Whole grain burger bun
Lettuce leaves, tomato slices, and red onion slices for serving

Instructions:

In a mixing bowl, combine lean ground turkey, chopped spinach leaves, crumbled feta cheese, minced garlic, salt, and pepper.
Form the mixture into a burger patty.
Grill the turkey burger patty over medium-high heat for 5-6 minutes on each side until cooked through.
Toast the whole grain burger bun until lightly golden.
Place the cooked turkey burger patty on the bottom half of the bun.
Top with lettuce leaves, tomato slices, and red onion slices.
Cover with the top half of the bun and serve immediately.

Nutritional Value (per serving)
Calories: 300 kcal
Protein: 25g
Fat: 10g
Carbohydrates: 30g
Fiber: 5g
Calcium: 8% DV
Vitamin D: 6% DV

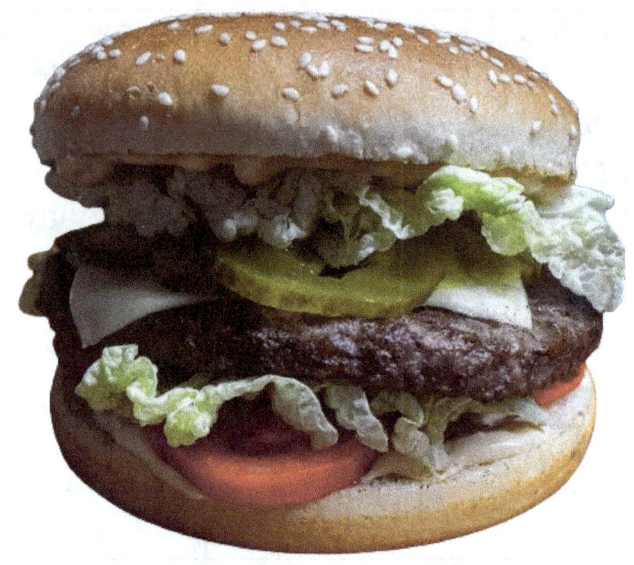

9. Veggie and Hummus Wrap
Ingredients:

1 large whole grain tortilla
2 tablespoons hummus
1/4 cup shredded carrots
1/4 cup sliced cucumbers
1/4 cup sliced bell peppers (assorted colors)
1/4 cup mixed greens (spinach, lettuce, arugula)
Salt and pepper to taste

Instructions:

Lay the whole grain tortilla flat on a clean surface.
Spread hummus evenly on the tortilla.
Layer shredded carrots, sliced cucumbers, sliced bell peppers, and mixed greens on top of the hummus.
Season with salt and pepper to taste.
Roll up the tortilla, tucking in the sides to enclose the filling.
Slice in half and serve immediately.

Nutritional Value (per serving)
Calories: 200 kcal
Protein: 6g
Fat: 8g
Carbohydrates: 25g
Fiber: 5g
Calcium: 6% DV
Vitamin D: 4% DV

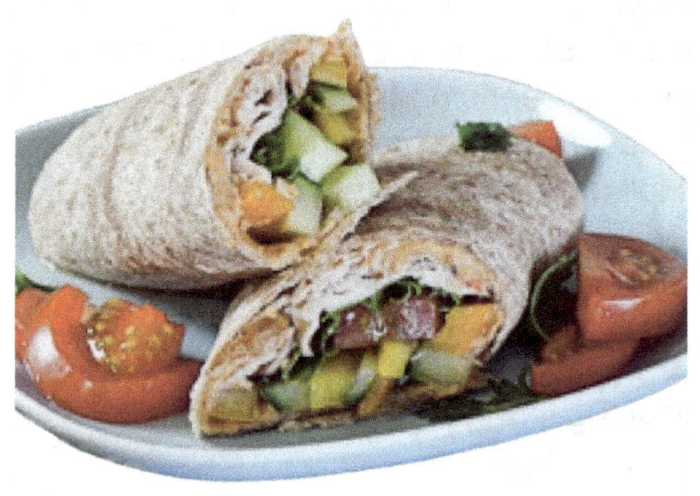

10. Mediterranean Chickpea Salad

Ingredients:

1 cup canned chickpeas, drained and rinsed
1/4 cup diced cucumber
1/4 cup diced tomatoes
1/4 cup diced red onion

2 tablespoons chopped fresh parsley
1 tablespoon extra virgin olive oil
1 tablespoon lemon juice
1/2 teaspoon dried oregano
Salt and pepper to taste
Crumbled feta cheese for garnish (optional)

Instructions:

In a mixing bowl, combine chickpeas, diced cucumber, diced tomatoes, diced red onion, chopped fresh parsley, extra virgin olive oil, lemon juice, dried oregano, salt, and pepper.

Toss until well combined.

Garnish with crumbled feta cheese if desired.

Serve chilled or at room temperature.

Nutritional Value (per serving)

Calories: 250 kcal

Protein: 10g

Fat: 10g

Carbohydrates: 30g

Fiber: 8g

Calcium: 8% DV

Vitamin D: 6% DV

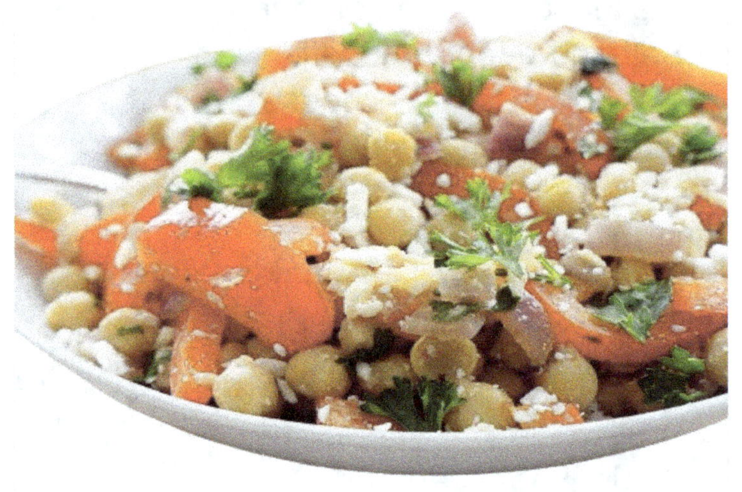

1. Baked Salmon with Roasted Vegetables

Ingredients:

4 oz salmon fillet

1 cup broccoli florets

1/2 cup cherry tomatoes

1/2 cup sliced bell peppers (assorted colors)

1/4 cup diced red onion
1 tablespoon olive oil
1 teaspoon minced garlic
Salt and pepper to taste
Lemon wedges for serving

Instructions:
Preheat the oven to 400°F (200°C).
Place salmon fillet on a baking sheet lined with parchment paper.
In a mixing bowl, toss broccoli florets, cherry tomatoes, sliced bell peppers, diced red onion, olive oil, minced garlic, salt, and pepper until well coated.
Spread the vegetable mixture around the salmon fillet on the baking sheet.
Bake for 15-20 minutes until the salmon is cooked through and the vegetables are tender.
Serve hot with lemon wedges.

Nutritional Value (per serving)
Calories: 300 kcal
Protein: 25g
Fat: 15g
Carbohydrates: 15g
Fiber: 5g

Calcium: 8% DV
Vitamin D: 15% DV

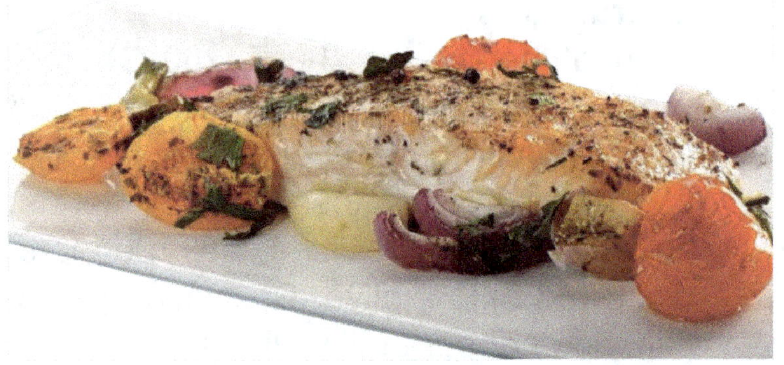

2. Quinoa and Black Bean Stuffed Peppers

Ingredients:

2 large bell peppers, halved and seeds removed

1 cup cooked quinoa

1/2 cup canned black beans, drained and rinsed

1/4 cup corn kernels

1/4 cup diced tomatoes

1/4 cup diced red onion

1/4 cup shredded cheddar cheese
1 tablespoon olive oil
1 teaspoon chili powder
Salt and pepper to taste
Fresh cilantro for garnish

Instructions:
Preheat the oven to 375°F (190°C).
In a large bowl, mix cooked quinoa, black beans, corn kernels, diced tomatoes, diced red onion, shredded cheddar cheese, olive oil, chili powder, salt, and pepper.
Stuff each bell pepper half with the quinoa mixture.
Place the stuffed bell peppers on a baking sheet lined with parchment paper.
Bake for 25-30 minutes until the peppers are tender and the filling is heated through.
Garnish with fresh cilantro before serving.

Nutritional Value (per serving, 1 stuffed pepper half)
Calories: 250 kcal

Protein: 10g
Fat: 8g
Carbohydrates: 35g
Fiber: 8g
Calcium: 10% DV
Vitamin D: 6% DV

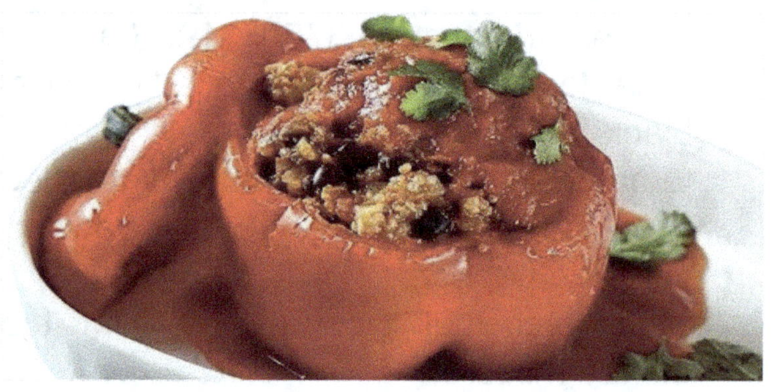

3. Chicken and Vegetable Skewers with Quinoa

Ingredients:

4 oz chicken breast, cubed
1/2 cup cherry tomatoes
1/2 cup bell peppers, cut into chunks (assorted colors)
1/2 cup zucchini, sliced
1/4 cup red onion, cut into chunks
1 tablespoon olive oil
1 teaspoon dried oregano

Salt and pepper to taste
1 cup cooked quinoa for serving

Instructions:
Preheat the grill or grill pan over medium-high heat.
In a mixing bowl, toss chicken breast cubes, cherry tomatoes, bell peppers, zucchini, red onion, olive oil, dried oregano, salt, and pepper until well coated.
Thread the marinated chicken and vegetables onto skewers.
Grill the skewers for 10-12 minutes, turning occasionally, until the chicken is cooked through and the vegetables are tender.
Serve hot with cooked quinoa.

Nutritional Value (per serving)
Calories: 350 kcal
Protein: 25g
Fat: 10g
Carbohydrates: 35g
Fiber: 6g
Calcium: 8% DV
Vitamin D: 6% DV

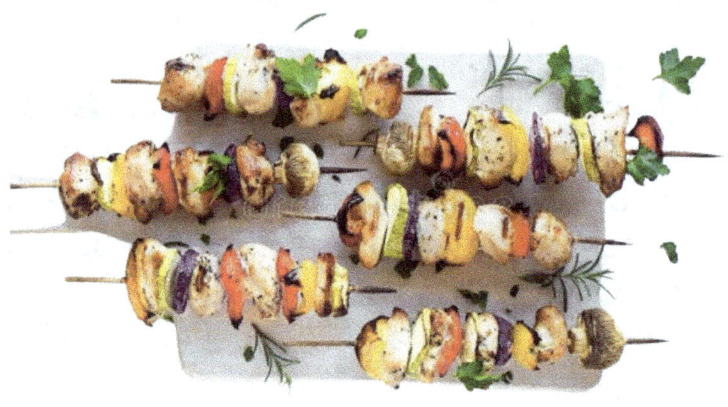

4. Spinach and Feta Stuffed Chicken Breast

Ingredients:

2 boneless, skinless chicken breasts
1 cup fresh spinach leaves
1/4 cup crumbled feta cheese
1 tablespoon olive oil
1 teaspoon minced garlic
Salt and pepper to taste
Lemon wedges for serving

Instructions:

Preheat the oven to 375°F (190°C).
Place chicken breasts on a cutting board and use a sharp knife to cut a slit horizontally along the side of each breast to form a pocket.
Stuff each chicken breast with fresh spinach leaves and crumbled feta cheese.
Season the stuffed chicken breasts with salt and pepper.
Heat olive oil in an oven-safe skillet over medium-high heat.
Add minced garlic to the skillet and cook for 1 minute until fragrant.
Add stuffed chicken breasts to the skillet and cook for 3-4 minutes on each side until browned.
Transfer the skillet to the preheated oven and bake for 20-25 minutes until the chicken is cooked through.
Serve hot with lemon wedges.

Nutritional Value (per serving)
Calories: 300 kcal
Protein: 30g
Fat: 15g
Carbohydrates: 5g

Fiber: 2g
Calcium: 8% DV
Vitamin D: 15% DV

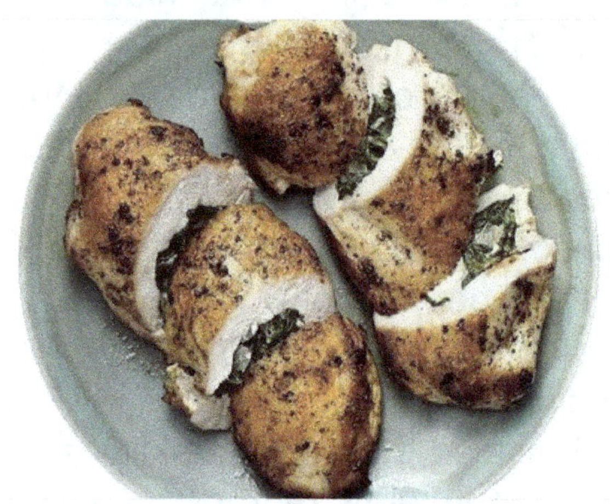

5. Lentil and Vegetable Curry
Ingredients:
1 cup dried lentils, rinsed and drained
2 cups vegetable broth
1 onion, diced
2 carrots, sliced
2 celery stalks, sliced
1 cup diced tomatoes
1 cup canned coconut milk
2 tablespoons curry powder
1 teaspoon minced garlic
Salt and pepper to taste
Fresh cilantro for garnish

Cooked brown rice for serving

Instructions:

In a large pot, combine dried lentils, vegetable broth, diced onion, sliced carrots, sliced celery, diced tomatoes, coconut milk, curry powder, minced garlic, salt, and pepper.

Bring the mixture to a boil over medium-high heat.

Reduce heat to low, cover, and simmer for 20-25 minutes until the lentils are tender and the vegetables are cooked through.

Serve hot over cooked brown rice.

Garnish with fresh cilantro before serving.

Nutritional Value (per serving)

Calories: 350 kcal
Protein: 15g
Fat: 10g
Carbohydrates: 50g
Fiber: 15g
Calcium: 6% DV
Vitamin D: 2% DV

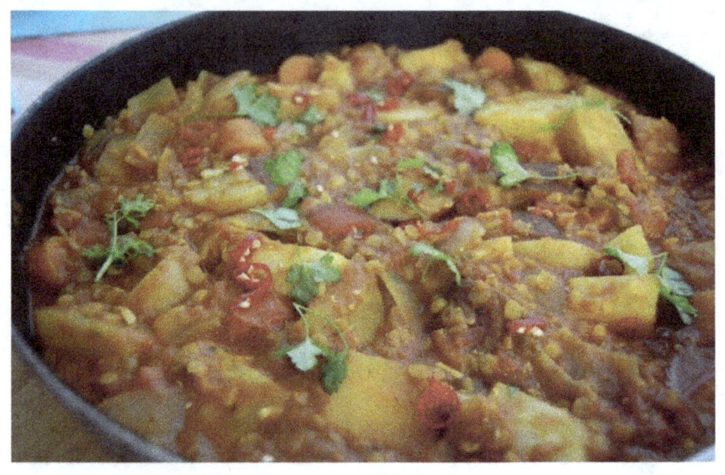

6. Turkey and Vegetable Stir-Fry
Ingredients:
4 oz lean ground turkey
1 cup broccoli florets
1/2 cup bell peppers, sliced (assorted colors)
1/2 cup snap peas
1/4 cup sliced carrots
1/4 cup diced onion
2 tablespoons low-sodium soy sauce
1 tablespoon olive oil
1 teaspoon minced garlic
1/2 teaspoon grated ginger
Sesame seeds for garnish (optional)
Cooked brown rice for serving

Instructions:

Heat olive oil in a large skillet or wok over medium-high heat.

Add minced garlic and grated ginger to the skillet and cook for 1 minute until fragrant.

Add lean ground turkey to the skillet and cook until browned.

Add broccoli florets, sliced bell peppers, snap peas, sliced carrots, and diced onion to the skillet and stir-fry until vegetables are tender-crisp.

Drizzle low-sodium soy sauce over the stir-fry and toss to coat.

Remove from heat and sprinkle with sesame seeds if desired.

Serve hot over cooked brown rice.

Nutritional Value (per serving)

Calories: 300 kcal

Protein: 20g

Fat: 10g

Carbohydrates: 30g

Fiber: 6g

Calcium: 6% DV

Vitamin D: 4% DV

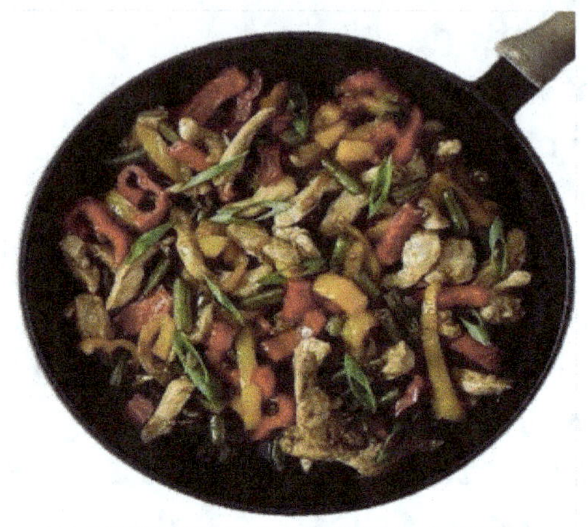

7. Spinach and Ricotta Stuffed shells

Ingredients:
8 oz jumbo pasta shells
1 cup ricotta cheese
1 cup chopped spinach leaves
1/4 cup grated Parmesan cheese
1 egg, lightly beaten
1 teaspoon minced garlic
Salt and pepper to taste
2 cups marinara sauce
Fresh basil leaves for garnish

Instructions:
Preheat the oven to 375°F (190°C).

Cook jumbo pasta shells according to package instructions until al dente. Drain and set aside.

In a mixing bowl, combine ricotta cheese, chopped spinach leaves, grated Parmesan cheese, lightly beaten egg, minced garlic, salt, and pepper.

Stuff each cooked pasta shell with the ricotta mixture.

Spread marinara sauce evenly in the bottom of a baking dish.

Arrange the stuffed pasta shells in the baking dish.

Cover with aluminum foil and bake for 25-30 minutes until heated through.

Remove foil and bake for an additional 5 minutes until cheese is melted and bubbly.

Garnish with fresh basil leaves before serving.

Nutritional Value (per serving)
Calories: 350 kcal
Protein: 20g
Fat: 15g
Carbohydrates: 35g
Fiber: 5g

Calcium: 15% DV
Vitamin D: 10% DV

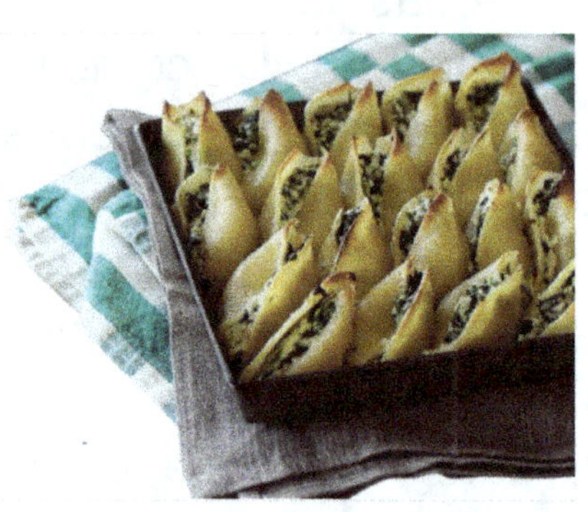

8. Vegetable and Tofu Stir-Fry
Ingredients:
8 oz extra-firm tofu, cubed
1 cup broccoli florets
1/2 cup bell peppers, sliced (assorted colors)
1/2 cup snap peas
1/4 cup sliced carrots
1/4 cup diced onion
2 tablespoons low-sodium soy sauce
1 tablespoon olive oil
1 teaspoon minced garlic
Salt and pepper to taste
Cooked brown rice for serving

Instructions:

Press tofu between paper towels to remove excess moisture. Cut tofu into cubes.

Heat olive oil in a large skillet or wok over medium-high heat.

Add minced garlic to the skillet and cook for 1 minute until fragrant.

Add tofu cubes to the skillet and cook until golden brown on all sides.

Add broccoli florets, sliced bell peppers, snap peas, sliced carrots, and diced onion to the skillet and stir-fry until vegetables are tender-crisp.

Drizzle low-sodium soy sauce over the stir-fry and toss to coat.

Remove from heat and season with salt and pepper to taste.

Serve hot over cooked brown rice.

Nutritional Value (per serving):
Calories: 300 kcal
Protein: 20g   Fat: 15g
Carbohydrates: 30g   Fiber: 6g
Calcium: 10% DV
Vitamin D: 4% DV

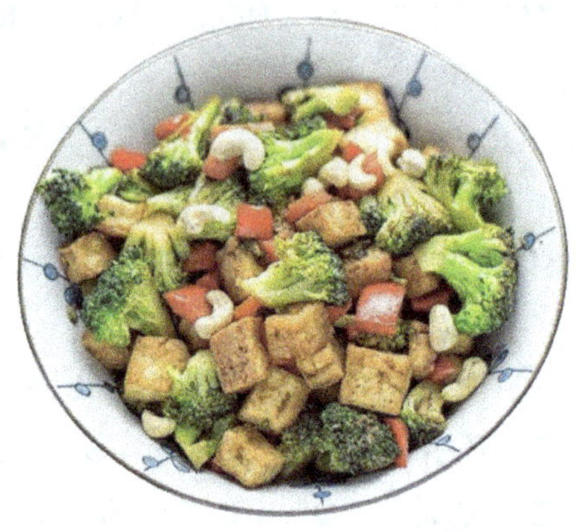

9. Baked Chicken Parmesan
Ingredients:
2 boneless, skinless chicken breasts
1/2 cup whole wheat breadcrumbs
1/4 cup grated Parmesan cheese
1 teaspoon dried Italian seasoning
1/2 cup marinara sauce
1/4 cup shredded mozzarella cheese
Fresh basil leaves for garnish
Cooked whole wheat pasta for serving

Instructions:
Preheat the oven to 375°F (190°C).
In a shallow dish, combine whole wheat
breadcrumbs, grated Parmesan cheese,
and dried Italian seasoning.

Coat each chicken breast with the breadcrumb mixture, pressing gently to adhere.
Place the coated chicken breasts on a baking sheet lined with parchment paper.
Bake for 20-25 minutes until the chicken is cooked through and the breadcrumbs are golden brown.
Remove from the oven and spoon marinara sauce evenly over each chicken breast.
Sprinkle shredded mozzarella cheese over the marinara sauce.
Return to the oven and bake for an additional 5 minutes until the cheese is melted and bubbly.
Garnish with fresh basil leaves before serving.
Serve hot with cooked whole wheat pasta.

Nutritional Value (per serving)

Calories: 350 kcal	Protein: 30g
Carbohydrates: 35g	Fat: 10g
Calcium: 15% DV	Fiber: 6g
Vitamin D: 10% DV	

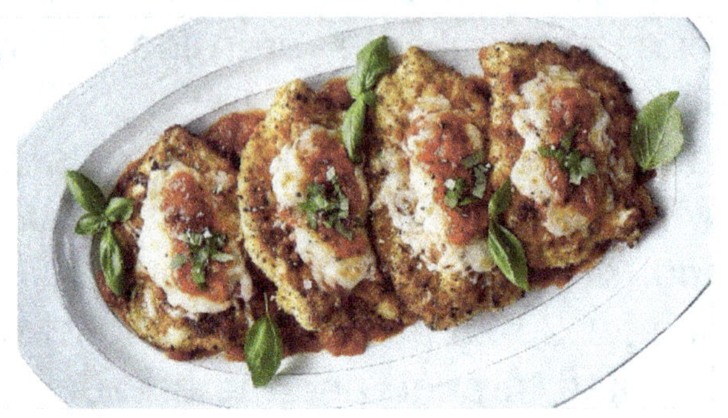

10. Vegetable and Lentil Soup
Ingredients:
1 cup dried lentils, rinsed and drained
4 cups vegetable broth
1 onion, diced
2 carrots, sliced
2 celery stalks, sliced
1 cup diced tomatoes
1 cup chopped spinach leaves
1 teaspoon dried thyme
1 teaspoon dried rosemary
Salt and pepper to taste
Fresh parsley for garnish

Instructions:

In a large pot, combine dried lentils, vegetable broth, diced onion, sliced

carrots, sliced celery, diced tomatoes, chopped spinach leaves, dried thyme, dried rosemary, salt, and pepper.
Bring the mixture to a boil over medium-high heat.
Reduce heat to low, cover, and simmer for 25-30 minutes until the lentils are tender and the vegetables are cooked through.
Season with salt and pepper to taste.
Ladle the soup into bowls and garnish with fresh parsley before serving.

Nutritional Value (per serving)
Calories: 250 kcal
Protein: 15g
Fat: 1g
Carbohydrates: 45g
Fiber: 15g
Calcium: 8% DV
Vitamin D: 2% DV

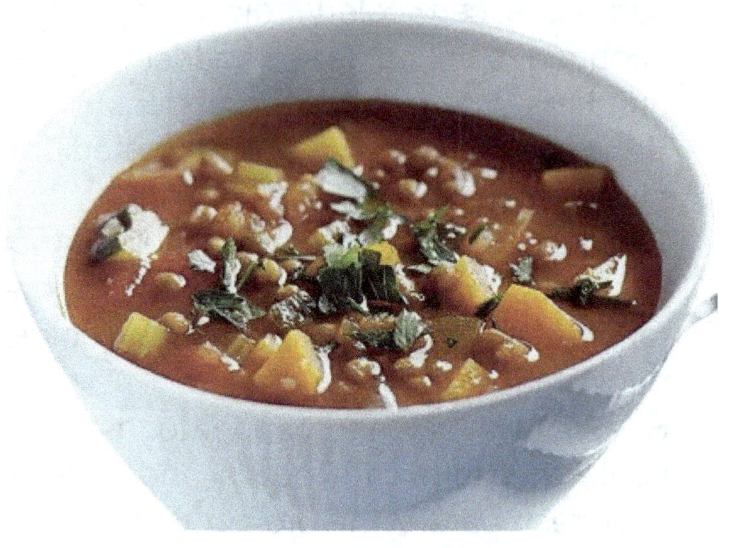

CONCLUSION

In concluding "The Osteoporosis Diet Cookbook for Women," it's evident that the journey towards optimal bone health is multifaceted and deeply intertwined with dietary choices. Throughout this comprehensive guide, we've explored the intricate relationship between nutrition and bone density, providing an arsenal of recipes and dietary strategies tailored specifically for women grappling with osteoporosis or aiming to prevent it.

One of the fundamental principles underscored in this cookbook is the importance of calcium intake. We've explored an array of calcium-rich foods, from dairy products to leafy greens, nuts, and fortified alternatives. Coupled with Vitamin D, these nutrients form the backbone of bone health, facilitating calcium absorption and ensuring the maintenance of bone density.

Moreover, I have highlighted the significance of protein in supporting bone structure and repair. The recipes presented have been crafted with a keen emphasis on incorporating lean protein sources, such as poultry, fish, beans, and legumes, into delicious and nutritionally balanced meals.

Furthermore, the role of micronutrients like magnesium, potassium, and vitamin K in bone metabolism has been thoroughly elucidated. By diversifying my culinary repertoire to include a spectrum of fruits, vegetables, and whole grains, we not only fortify our bones but also nurture overall health and vitality.

Beyond mere nutritional recommendations, this cookbook has also addressed lifestyle factors crucial for bone health. From the imperative of regular weight-bearing exercises to the significance of adequate hydration and the perils of excessive alcohol and caffeine consumption, holistic approaches to osteoporosis management have been underscored.

Importantly, "The Osteoporosis Diet Cookbook for Women" does not merely offer a compendium of recipes; it serves as a guide to empowerment and proactive health management. By fostering a deeper understanding of the intricacies of bone health and the pivotal role of nutrition therein, readers are equipped to make informed choices that resonate throughout their lives.

In essence, this cookbook contains a holistic approach to bone health, merging culinary creativity with evidence-based dietary strategies and lifestyle modifications. As readers embark on their culinary adventures armed with this knowledge, they embark on a journey towards fortified bones, enhanced well-being, and a zestful life. May each recipe shared within these pages serve not only to nourish the body but also to nurture a sense of empowerment and vitality for all women navigating the terrain of osteoporosis.

THANK YOU FOR GETTING ONE FOR YOURSELF, DO WELL TO GET FOR YOUR LOVED ONES TOO.

Love From the writer
Dr. Samantha Hayes